A Kid's Guide to Vitamins and Minerals

Preface

'A Kid's Guide to Vitamins and Minerals' is bound to serve as invaluable guide for students or any other person who wants to know about the basic information regarding Vitamins and Minerals required by our body in an easy language.

The book contains attractive pictures which are bound to captivate young readers. The book contains two chapters divided into different sections and a separate chapter is devoted towards Vitamin D.

The author hopes that this book will serve its purpose of spreading knowledge in a simplified manner.

Copyright

Table of Content

Chapter1: Vitamins

WHAT ARE VITAMINS?

Vitamins are complex organic chemicals that our present in our food in small quantities. Vitamins are essential for growth, good health, proper vision, normal digestion process and synchronised activities of our body. Vitamins are essential for growth, good health, proper vision, normal digestion process, etc.

CLASSIFICATION OF VITAMINS

According to their solubility in either fat or water, vitamins can be classified into two types-

1. FAT-SOLUBLE VITAMINS

The vitamins which are soluble in fats are called fat-soluble vitamins. They occur in foods containing fats and are stored in the body either in the liver or in the fatty tissues. Vitamins A, D, E and K are fat-soluble vitamins.

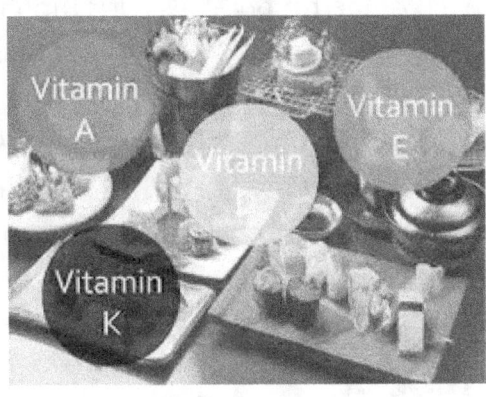

2. WATER-SOLUBLE VITAMINS

Vitamins which are soluble in water are called water-soluble vitamins. They are not stored in our body and excess is excreted out in the urine. Vitamin C and B are water-soluble vitamins.

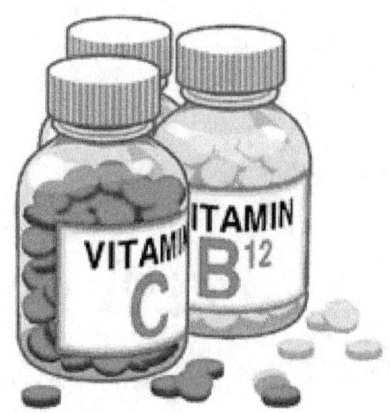

<u>DIFFERENCE TABLE</u>

	Water Soluble	Fat Soluble
Absorption	Directly into the blood	First into the lymph node, then the blood
Transport	Travel Freely	May require protein carriers

Toxicity	Possible to reach toxic levels due to the excess consumption of supplements	Can reach toxic levels due to excess consumption of supplements
Excretion	Excess is remove through urine	Stored in fat storage tissues

FUNCTIONS OR IMPORTANCE OF VITAMINS

FAT-SOLUBLE VITAMINS
Vitamin-A
SCIENTIFIC NAME- RETINOL

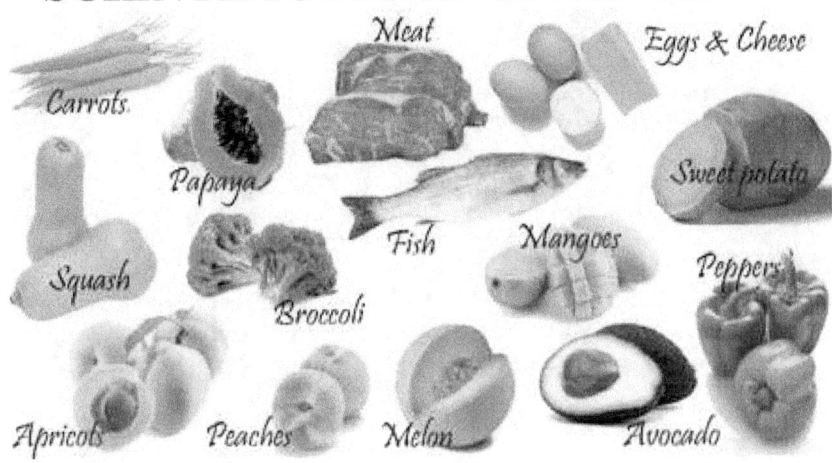

1. Promotes Growth.
2. Helps to maintain proper vision.
3. Essential for healthy skin and other body tissues.
4. Keeps the teeth structure healthy.

Deficiency Disease- Night Blindness

FOOD SOURCES-EGGS, MILK, CREAM, CHEESE, LIVER, GREEN AND YELLOW VEGETABLES AND CARROTS, SWEET POTATOES, SPINACH, FISH, RIPE MANGOES

VITAMIN-D
SCIENTIFIC NAME-
CALCIFEROL

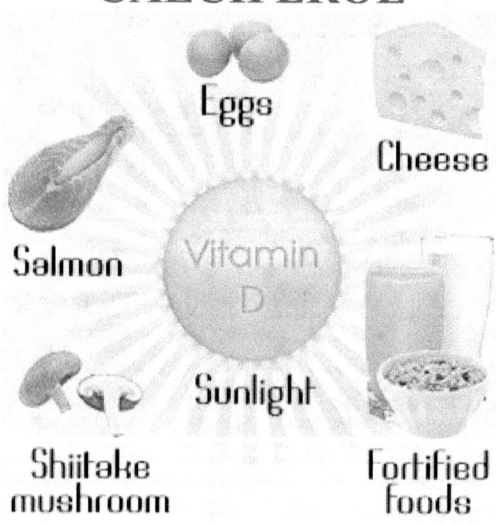

1. Essential for maintaining calcium and phosphorus levels in the body by enhancing their absorption in the intestine.
2. Helps in regulating exchange between blood and bones.

Deficiency Disease- Rickets

FOOD SOURCES- MILK, BUTTER, FISH, COD LIVER OIL, EGGS AND SUNLIGHT

VITAMIN-E
SCIENTIFIC NAME- TOCOPHEROL

Sources of Vitamin E

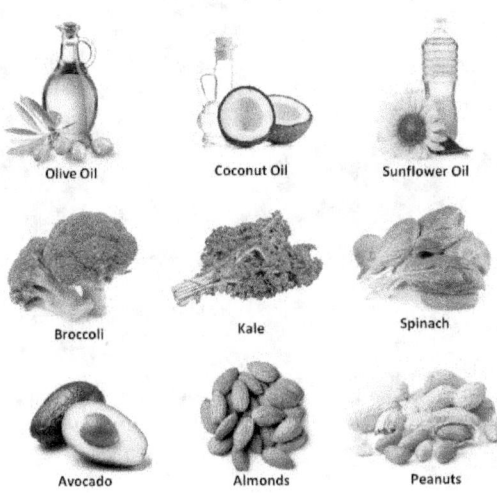

1. Essential for nutrition.
2. Associated with intake of polyunsaturated fatty acids.

Deficiency Disease- Growth and Fertility Disorders

FOOD SOURCES- EGG YOLK, CEREALS, LIVER, MILK, BUTTER, WHEAT GERM OIL, GREEN LEAFY VEGETABLES

VITAMIN-K SCIENTIFIC NAME- PHYLLOQUINONE

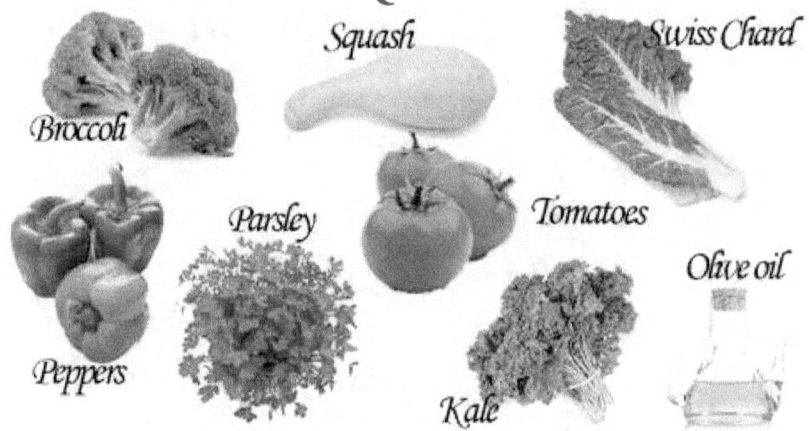

Essential for the normal clotting of blood.

Deficiency Disease- Delayed Blood Clotting and Haemorrhage

FOOD SOURCES- GREEN LEAFY VEGETABLES, LIVER, SOYA BEAN AND TOMATOES

WATER-SOLUBLE VITAMINS
VITAMIN-B1
SCIENTIFIC NAME- THIAMINE

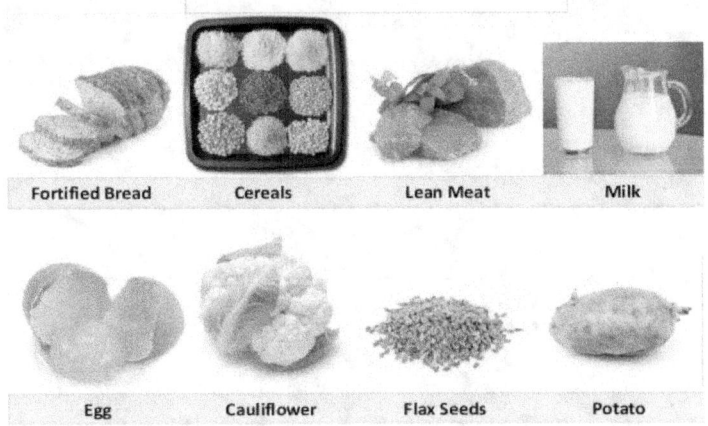

Sources of Vitamin B1

Fortified Bread · Cereals · Lean Meat · Milk

Egg · Cauliflower · Flax Seeds · Potato

1. Helps in carbohydrate metabolism.
2. Normal functioning of heart, nerves and muscles.

Deficiency Disease- Beri Beri

FOOD SOURCES- MILK, SEAFOOD, MEAT, LIVER, YEAST, WHOLE GREEN CEREALS AND GREEN VEGETABLES

VITAMIN-B2
SCIENTIFIC NAME- RIBOFLAVIN

1. Regulates food oxidation.
2. Acts as a key component in certain enzymes.

**DEFICIENCY DISEASE-
ARIBOFLAVINOSIS**

FOOD SOURCES- MILK, PEAS, BEANS,
MEAT, EGGS, CEREALS (WHOLE GRAIN),
GREEN LEAFY VEGETABLES AND YEAST

VITAMIN-B3
SCIENTIFIC NAME- NIACIN

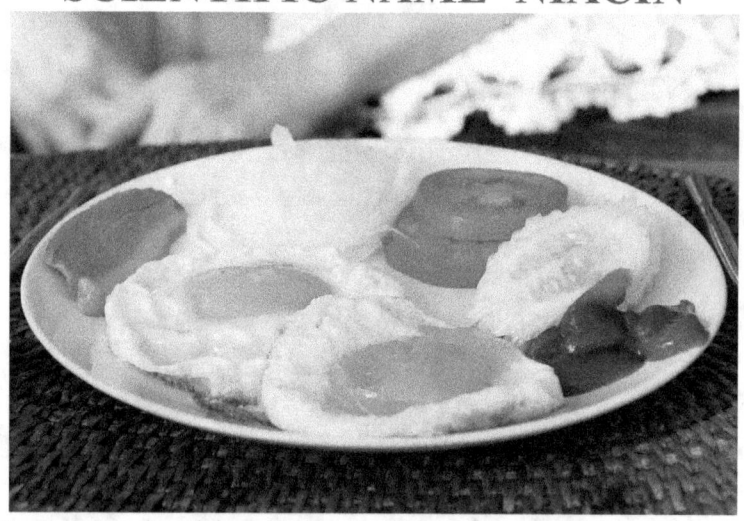

Promotes health of skin and nervous system.

DEFICIENCY SYSTEM- PELLAGRA

FOOD SOURCES- PEANUTS, MEAT,
POULTRY, LIVER, FISH, BRAN, YEAST,
WHOLE GRAINS, TOMATO, POTATO

VITAMIN-B11
SCIENTIFIC NAME- FOLIC ACID

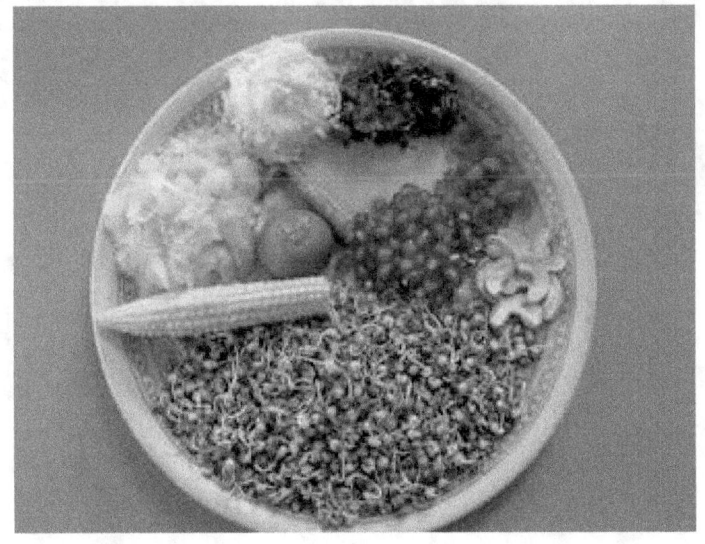

1. Essential for formation and maturation of RBCs.
2. Required to form DNA.

DEFICIENCY DISEASE- PERINICIOUS ANAEMIA

FOOD SOURCES- GREEN LEAFY
VEGETABLES, SPROUTED PULSES

VITAMIN-B12
SCIENTIFIC NAME-
COBALAMIN

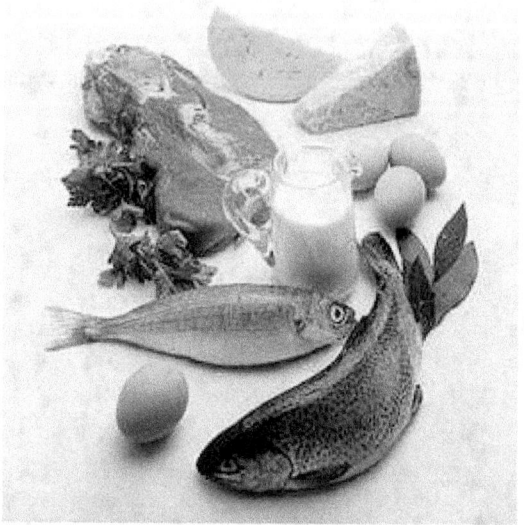

Essential for nucleic acid synthesis in rapidly dividing cells.

DEFICIENCY DISEASE- ANAEMIA

FOOD SOURCES- EGGS, MILK, LEVER, MEAT

VITAMIN-C
SCIENTIFIC NAME- ASCORBIC
ACID

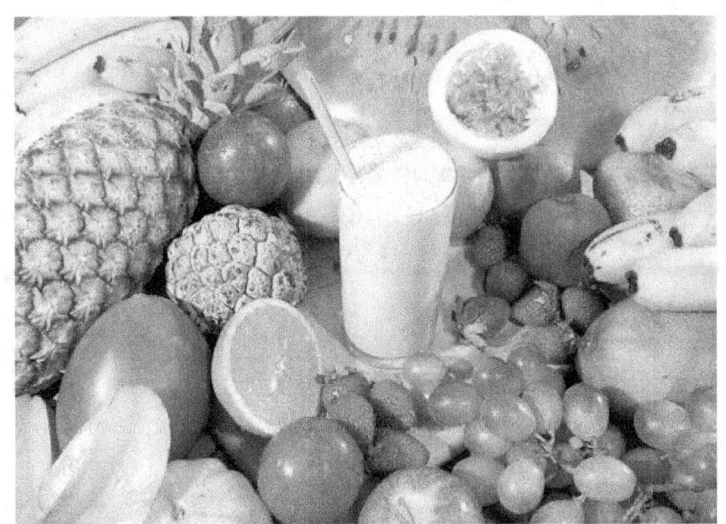

Essential for maintenance of connective tissue.

DEFICIENCY DISEASE- SCURVY

FOOD SOURCES- FRESH CITRUS FRUITS LIKE ORANGE, AMLA, LIME, LEMON, GUAVA, TOMATO, GOOSEBERRY, CABBAGE

Chapter 2: Minerals

DEFINITION OF MINERALS

A mineral is an inorganic element, occurring in the form of its salt, e.g. Calcium, potassium, sodium, phosphorus, iron, copper, magnesium, etc.

CLASSIFICATION OF MINERALS

Depending on their functions, minerals required by our body can be classified into 2 categories-

1. MAJOR MINERALS OR MACROMINERALS

These minerals are needed in relatively large amounts in our diet i.e. over 100 mg (milligram) per day; examples are- sodium, sulphur, chloride, potassium and magnesium.

2. TRACE MINERALS OR TRACE ELEMENTS

These minerals are needed in smaller amounts, i.e. only a few mg (milligrams) per day in our diet; examples are- copper, zinc, fluoride, manganese, iodine, fluoride and cobalt.

Functions of Minerals and Their Food Sources

CALCIUM

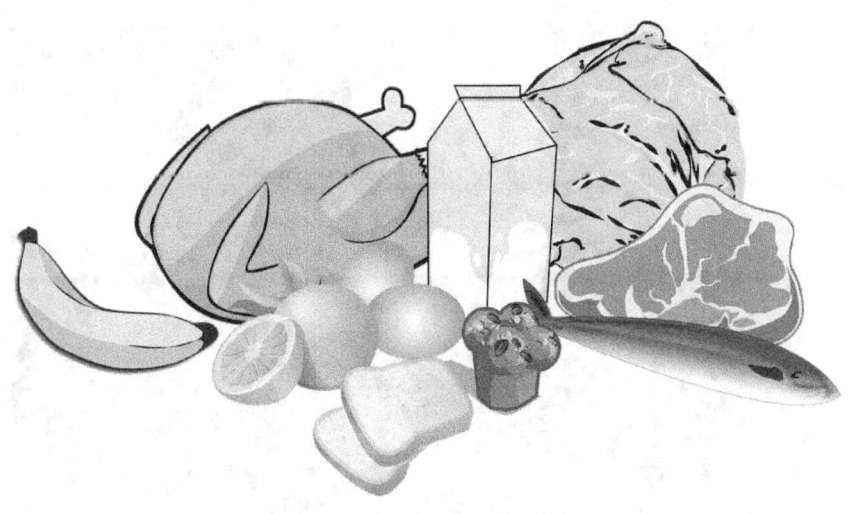

1. Helps in the formation of bones and teeth.
2. Helps in blood clotting.
3. Helps in muscle contraction.
4. Helps in nerve impulse transmission.

DEFICINECY- MEMORY LOSS, HALLUCINATION, BONE PAIN AND CONFUSION

FOOD SOURCES- MILK AND MILK PRODUCTS, BROCCOLI, BEANS, GREEN VEGETABLES, WHOLE GRAM, CEREALS, MEAT, FISH AND TAPIOCA

PHOSPHORUS

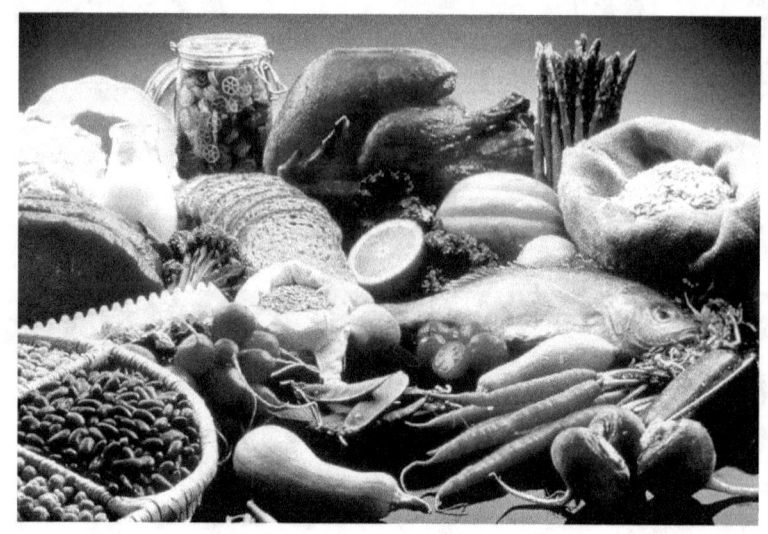

1. Helps in the formation of bones and teeth.
2. Helps in the formation of DNA.
3. Helps in the formation of many enzymes.

DEFICIENCY- FATIGUE, BONE OAIN, STIFF JOINTS, WEAKNESS, NUMBNESS, LOSS OF APPETITE AND IRRITABILITY

FOOD SOURCES- MILK AND MILK PRODUCTS, MEAT, POULTRY, BAJRA, NUTS, FISH, EGGS, LIVER AND KIDNEY

POTASSIUM

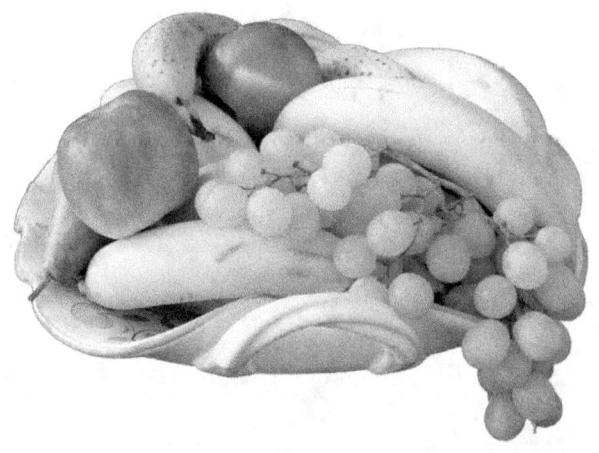

1. Keeps the water and acid-base (electrolyte) balance.
2. Helps in muscle contraction.
3. Helps in nerve impulse transaction.

DEFICIENCY- CONSTIPATION AND FATIGUE

FOOD SOURCES- MILK, YOGHURT, ORANGES, PEAS, POTATOES

SODIUM

1. Keeps the water and acid base balance.
2. Helps in the contraction of muscles.
3. Assists in the transmission of nerve impulse.

DEFICIENCY- HYPONATREMIA, GASTROINTESTINAL PROBLEMS AND MUSCULAR PROBLEMS
FOOD SOURCES- COMMON SALT, FISH, PICKLES, MEAT, EGGS, FAST FOODS

IRON

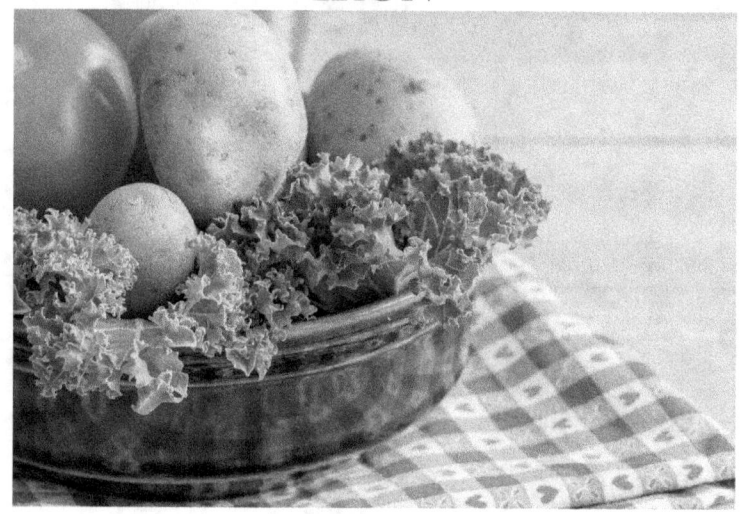

1. Essential for normal metabolism.
2. Helps in the formation of haemoglobin and myoglobin.
3. Important part of some enzymes.
4. Helps in the energy metabolism and formation of new cells.
5. Helps in tissue Oxidation.

DEFICIENCY- TIREDNESS, DIZZINESS

AND HEAVY BREATHING

FOOD SOURCES- LIVER, KIDNEY, EGGS, MEAT, GROUNDNUT, CEREALS, GREEN LEAFY VEGETABLES, LEGUMES, SPINACH

IODINE

Helps in the proper functioning of Thyroid Gland (for secretion of thyroxin).

DEFICIENCY- GOITRE

FOOD SOURCES- IODISED SALT, SALT-WATER FISH, SEA FOOD, GREEN LEAFY VEGETABLES

Chapter 3: Vitamin D Guide

Vitamin D also known as Calciferol is essential for maintaining the calcium and phosphorus levels in the body by enhancing their absorption in the intestine and regulating exchange between blood and bones. Helps to keep teeth and bones healthy and makes the immune system stronger.

HOW OUR SKIN SYNTHESIS VITAMIN D?

Vitamin D is synthesised when the bare skin is exposed the ultraviolet B (UVB) rays. Most people get the recommended amount of sunlight to produce Vitamin D.

FACTORS AFFECTING VITAMIN D FORMATION IN OUR BODY

Factors determining the Vitamin D production are-

1. **Age-** Young people produce more Vitamin D as compared to old people.
2. **Skin Color-** More darker the skin color (More the Melanin) less will the skin's chances to absorb UVB rays. Therefore Dark Skinned People need to sunbath as compared to White Skinned People.
3. **Time Period to which the skin is exposed to the Sun.**

4. **Season-** During Winters the skin needs to be exposed more to the sunlight.
5. **Country-** The latitude in which the country is situated has an influence on th UVB rays of the Sun reaching the Earth.
6. **Sunscreen Lotions and Clothing-** Sunscreen lotions applied on the skin or the level of clothing greatly influences our skin's ability to absorb the UVB rays.
7. **Obesity-** Science proves that obese persons have difficulty to convert the UVB rays into Vitamin D.
8. **Weight-** The more fat a person has the more Vitamin D will help in the storage in the storage of nutrients however obesity reduces the formation of Vitamin D.

SYMPTOMS OF VITAMIN D DEFICIENCY

Bone pain, muscle pain and brittleness, dark skin pigmentation and overweight are the symptoms of Vitamin D Deficiency. According to medical reports more than 25 to 50% population may be suffering from Vitamin D deficiency.